MAGNESIUM MIRACLES

The Gateway of Optimal Health

Katherine Peters

Copyright © 2024 by [Katherine Peters]

All rights reserved. No part of this book may be reproduced in any form or by any electronic or mechanical means, including information storage and retrieval systems, without permission in writing from the publisher, except by a reviewer who may quote brief passages in a review.

The information in this book is for educational purposes only. It is not intended to diagnose, treat, cure, or prevent any disease or medical condition. The author and publisher are not responsible for any adverse effects or consequences resulting from the use of the information contained in this book.

Table of Contents

Part I: Understanding Magnesium

Introduction
Overview of Magnesium

Chapter One
The Crucial Role of Magnesium in Human Health

Chapter Two
The Science Behind Magnesium: Essential Functions Explained

Part II: Health Benefits of Magnesium

Chapter Three
Guarding Against Heart Disease with Magnesium

Chapter Four
Magnesium and Brain Health: Alleviating Depression, Anxiety, and More

Chapter Five
Magnesium for Joint Health: Easing Arthritis and Inflammation

Chapter Six

Respiratory Health and Asthma: How Magnesium Helps

Part III: Magnesium in Daily Life

Chapter Seven
Understanding Magnesium Deficiency: Causes and Signs

Chapter Eight
Maximizing Magnesium Intake: Dietary Sources and Supplements

Chapter Nine
Enhancing Absorption: Optimizing Your Body's Utilization of Magnesium

Part IV: Lifestyle and Beyond

Chapter Ten
The Role of Magnesium in Stress Reduction and Sleep Enhancement

Chapter Eleven
Physical Activity and Magnesium: How Exercise Affects Levels

Chapter Twelve
Embracing the Magnesium Miracle: Actionable Steps for a Healthier Life

Part I: Understanding Magnesium

Introduction

Overview of Magnesium

A fundamental component of human health and vigor, magnesium is an elemental mineral that is necessary for life. This basic but essential mineral, which is widely distributed in nature, plays a part in almost every area of human physiological function.

Magnesium: Nature's Vital Element

The Elemental Foundation

Magnesium, which has the atomic number 12 and the chemical symbol Mg, is an essential component of more than 300 enzymatic processes in the human body. It serves as a catalyst in cellular energy production, DNA synthesis, and the regulation of diverse biochemical processes that sustain life.

Nature's Magnesium Reservoir

Magnesium is widely distributed throughout the Earth's crust and can be found in a variety of forms. The main sources of magnesium for human intake include saltwater, mineral deposits, and specific foods. Rich food sources of magnesium include whole grains, legumes, nuts, seeds, and green leafy vegetables. Supplemental magnesium is another way to be sure you're getting enough of it.

The Magnesium Equilibrium

Despite its critical relevance, magnesium shortage affects a large number of people in a variety of demographics, including those living in industrialized countries. This widespread deficiency is a result of a number of factors, including poor food choices, soil erosion, stress, excessive alcohol or caffeine usage, and some drugs.

The Vital Connection to Human Health

Heart-related Conditions
A healthy cardiovascular system is greatly dependent on magnesium. It helps to control blood pressure, maintains blood vessel health, and controls heart rhythm. Its ability to lower the risk of heart disease and stroke is highlighted by research.

Bone Health

Magnesium is essential to bone structure and works in tandem with calcium to preserve bone strength and density. It may help maintain the health and function of muscles while lowering the risk of osteoporosis and bone fractures.

Harmony of Metabolic Processes

Magnesium affects glucose metabolism and insulin sensitivity, making it a crucial component of metabolism. By controlling blood sugar levels and reducing insulin resistance, it helps treat diabetes.

Mental Health

The mineral exhibits a significant effect on neurotransmitter activity and mood modulation, hence altering mental health. Research indicates that it may help reduce stress, anxiety, and depressive symptoms.

Moving Forward: Accepting the Magnesium Miracle

Closing the Deficiency Distance

The importance of magnesium insufficiency makes it imperative to implement measures to guarantee appropriate consumption. This means accepting dietary adjustments, investigating supplementation under supervision, and reducing conditions that cause the body to lose magnesium reserves.

Chapter One

The Crucial Role of Magnesium in Human Health

Magnesium, often dubbed the "forgotten mineral," plays a pivotal role in orchestrating an array of essential bodily functions. Its presence and participation are fundamental to numerous physiological processes, spanning from cellular energy production to the regulation of enzymatic reactions, and far beyond.

Cellular Energy Production

At the heart of cellular energy metabolism lies magnesium. It acts as a catalyst in the synthesis of adenosine triphosphate (ATP), the body's primary energy currency. Without sufficient magnesium, cells struggle to produce the energy required for various biological activities, resulting in fatigue and diminished vitality.

Enzymatic Reactions and Biochemical Processes

Magnesium serves as a cofactor in over 300 enzymatic reactions, facilitating diverse biochemical processes crucial for maintaining homeostasis. It contributes to DNA and RNA synthesis, protein formation, and the modulation of neurotransmitters and hormones, underscoring its pervasive influence.

Muscle Function and Relaxation

Crucial for neuromuscular function, magnesium aids in muscle contraction and relaxation. It plays a role in calcium transport across cell membranes, regulating muscle contractions and preventing excessive muscle tension or spasms.

Cardiovascular Health and Blood Pressure Regulation

The mineral exerts a profound influence on cardiovascular well-being. It supports heart rhythm regulation, helps maintain healthy blood vessel function, and contributes to blood pressure control. Magnesium deficiency has been linked to increased risks of heart disease, arrhythmias, and hypertension.

Bone Strength and Density

Magnesium collaborates with calcium and other minerals to uphold skeletal integrity. It enhances calcium absorption and deposition in bones, contributing to bone density and strength.

Insufficient magnesium levels may compromise bone health and increase the risk of osteoporosis.

Metabolic Harmony and Insulin Sensitivity

Critical for metabolic processes, magnesium influences insulin sensitivity, glucose regulation, and carbohydrate metabolism. Adequate magnesium levels assist in insulin signaling, contributing to improved glycemic control and reduced risk of insulin resistance.

Neurological Health and Mood Regulation

The mineral's involvement in neurotransmitter regulation, particularly in the brain, underscores its significance in mood regulation, stress management, and cognitive function. Studies suggest its potential in mitigating symptoms of depression, anxiety, and stress

Chapter Two

The Science Behind Magnesium: Essential Functions Explained

Magnesium, a remarkable mineral with multifaceted roles in human physiology, operates as a key player in countless biological processes, owing to its chemical properties and interactions within the body.

Atomic Structure and Bioavailability

As an alkaline earth metal, magnesium (Mg) stands as the eighth most abundant element in the Earth's crust. Its atomic structure, comprising 12 protons, 12 electrons, and 12 neutrons, contributes to its stability and reactivity. In biological systems, magnesium primarily exists in its ionized form (Mg^{2+}), crucial for its bioavailability and functionality.

Enzymatic Reactions and ATP Synthesis

Magnesium acts as a cofactor in enzymatic reactions, facilitating their catalytic functions. Particularly vital is its role in adenosine triphosphate (ATP) synthesis within the mitochondria, the cellular powerhouses. ATP, the body's energy currency, relies on magnesium for its formation, making magnesium an indispensable component in cellular energy production.

Structural Integrity and DNA Synthesis

Beyond its enzymatic roles, magnesium contributes to maintaining structural integrity within cells. It assists in the stabilization of DNA and RNA, supporting their synthesis and aiding in the transmission of genetic information. Magnesium's presence ensures the fidelity of genetic replication and protein synthesis.

Ion Transport and Cellular Signaling

Magnesium's influence extends to ion transport across cell membranes, regulating the influx and efflux of various ions, notably calcium. This interplay between magnesium and calcium is integral to cellular signaling, muscle contraction, and nerve impulse transmission, ensuring the delicate balance between excitation and relaxation in cells.

Cardiovascular Modulation and Blood Pressure Regulation

Within the cardiovascular system, magnesium plays a pivotal role in maintaining heart rhythm and vascular tone. It facilitates the relaxation of blood vessel walls, thereby regulating blood pressure. Additionally, magnesium aids in mitigating inflammation, oxidative stress, and endothelial dysfunction, promoting cardiovascular health.

Metabolic Regulation and Insulin Sensitivity

In metabolic pathways, magnesium influences insulin signaling and glucose metabolism. It aids in insulin-mediated glucose uptake by cells, fostering improved insulin sensitivity. This mechanism supports glycemic control, mitigating the risk of insulin resistance and type 2 diabetes.

Neurological Function and Neurotransmitter Regulation

The mineral's impact on the nervous system involves neurotransmitter release, nerve impulse transmission, and mood regulation. Magnesium modulates neurotransmitter activity, including serotonin, promoting emotional balance and stress resilience.

Part II: Health Benefits of Magnesium

Chapter Three

Guarding Against Heart Disease with Magnesium

Heart disease remains a leading cause of mortality globally, prompting a deeper exploration into the potential benefits of magnesium in fortifying cardiovascular health. Research suggests that magnesium, an often-overlooked mineral, plays a crucial role in mitigating the risk factors associated with heart disease.

Blood Pressure Regulation

Magnesium contributes significantly to maintaining healthy blood pressure levels. It aids in the relaxation of blood vessels, reducing resistance to blood flow and assisting in the regulation of arterial pressure. Studies indicate that adequate magnesium intake correlates with lower blood pressure, thus reducing the risk of hypertension—a significant precursor to heart disease.

Rhythm Regulation and Arrhythmia Prevention

The mineral's role in regulating heart rhythm stands as a critical aspect of cardiovascular health. Magnesium ensures the proper functioning of ion channels within cardiac cells, influencing the electrical impulses that coordinate heartbeats. Adequate magnesium levels may help prevent arrhythmias and irregular heartbeats, thus reducing the risk of cardiac complications.

Anti-inflammatory and Vasodilatory Effects

Magnesium exhibits anti-inflammatory properties that benefit heart health. By mitigating inflammation and oxidative stress, magnesium helps protect the endothelium—the lining of blood vessels—promoting its proper function. Additionally, magnesium acts as a natural vasodilator, aiding in the relaxation of blood vessels and enhancing blood flow.

LDL Cholesterol Regulation

Emerging research suggests that magnesium plays a role in regulating LDL cholesterol (the "bad" cholesterol) levels. Adequate magnesium intake has been associated with lower LDL cholesterol and triglyceride levels, potentially reducing the risk of atherosclerosis and plaque formation within arterial walls.

Antithrombotic Effects

Magnesium demonstrates antithrombotic properties, contributing to blood clot prevention. By modulating platelet aggregation and clot formation, magnesium reduces the likelihood of thrombotic events that can lead to heart attacks or strokes.

Chapter Four

Magnesium and Brain Health: Alleviating Depression, Anxiety, and More

Beyond its well-documented roles in physiological functions, magnesium showcases a profound influence on brain health and mental well-being. Its involvement in neurotransmitter regulation, neuronal signaling, and stress modulation underscores its significance in addressing conditions such as depression, anxiety, and cognitive decline.

Neurotransmitter Regulation and Mood Enhancement

Magnesium plays a pivotal role in neurotransmitter regulation, affecting the release and activity of neurotransmitters such as serotonin—a key player in mood regulation. Adequate magnesium levels contribute to enhanced serotonin synthesis and availability, promoting a balanced mood and potentially alleviating symptoms of depression and anxiety.

Stress Mitigation and Cortisol Regulation

Magnesium acts as a natural stress buffer by modulating the hypothalamic-pituitary-adrenal (HPA) axis—a central component of the body's stress response. By regulating cortisol levels, magnesium aids in mitigating the physiological effects of stress, thereby reducing the likelihood of stress-related mental health conditions.

Cognitive Function and Memory Enhancement

Research suggests that magnesium plays a role in cognitive function and memory consolidation. Its involvement in neuronal signaling pathways and synaptic plasticity—critical components of learning and memory—positions magnesium as a potential ally in supporting cognitive health and potentially mitigating age-related cognitive decline.

Anxiety Reduction and Nervous System Support

Magnesium's calming effects on the nervous system contribute to anxiety reduction. By modulating neuronal excitability and promoting GABA (gamma-aminobutyric acid) function—a neurotransmitter that fosters relaxation—magnesium aids in reducing symptoms of anxiety and promoting a sense of calmness.

Sleep Quality Improvement

Optimal magnesium levels have been linked to improved sleep quality. Magnesium supports the regulation of melatonin—a hormone crucial for sleep-wake cycles—enhancing sleep duration and quality. Adequate magnesium intake may aid in addressing sleep disturbances and insomnia.

Chapter Five

Magnesium for Joint Health: Easing Arthritis and Inflammation

Often lauded for its involvement in various physiological functions, magnesium, extends its influence to joint health, offering potential relief for individuals grappling with arthritis and inflammatory conditions affecting the joints.

Anti-inflammatory Properties

Magnesium showcases remarkable anti-inflammatory properties, critical in managing joint-related conditions characterized by inflammation, such as rheumatoid arthritis and osteoarthritis. By modulating inflammatory pathways and cytokine production, magnesium aids in reducing joint swelling, stiffness, and pain.

Calcium Balance and Joint Protection

In tandem with calcium, magnesium contributes to maintaining proper bone density and joint integrity. Its interaction with calcium ensures a balanced ratio between these minerals, thereby safeguarding against calcium deposition in joints—an occurrence associated with arthritis and joint degeneration.

Muscle Relaxation and Pain Reduction

Magnesium's role in muscle relaxation is particularly beneficial for individuals experiencing joint discomfort. By aiding in muscle relaxation and alleviating muscle tension, magnesium indirectly mitigates stress on the joints, potentially reducing pain and discomfort associated with conditions like arthritis.

Cartilage Health and Protection

Studies indicate that magnesium plays a role in supporting cartilage health—a vital component of joint structure. It contributes to collagen synthesis, aiding in the preservation of cartilage integrity and potentially slowing down joint degeneration.

Symptom Management and Functionality Improvement

Incorporating adequate magnesium levels into one's diet or through supplementation may assist in managing the symptoms of arthritis, promoting better joint functionality, and enhancing mobility. Magnesium's anti-inflammatory effects coupled with its influence on muscle relaxation contribute to improved joint comfort and movement.

The anti-inflammatory, muscle-relaxant, and cartilage-supporting properties of magnesium render it a promising adjunct in managing joint-related conditions, including arthritis and inflammation. Incorporating magnesium-rich foods or supplements may offer relief, improve joint functionality, and potentially alleviate discomfort associated with joint conditions, promoting a better quality of life for individuals grappling with joint health issues.

Chapter Six

Respiratory Health and Asthma: How Magnesium Helps

Magnesium, renowned for its multifaceted roles in physiological functions, extends its influence to respiratory health, showcasing potential benefits in mitigating symptoms associated with asthma and supporting overall lung function.

Bronchodilation and Airway Relaxation

Magnesium exhibits bronchodilatory properties, aiding in airway relaxation and expansion. For individuals with asthma—a condition characterized by airway constriction and inflammation—magnesium's ability to dilate bronchi may offer relief by easing breathing difficulties and reducing the severity of asthma attacks.

Anti-inflammatory Effects and Asthma Management

The mineral's anti-inflammatory properties play a crucial role in managing asthma-related inflammation. Magnesium modulates inflammatory pathways, potentially reducing airway inflammation and mucus production, thereby alleviating asthma symptoms and promoting easier breathing.

Improved Lung Function and Respiratory Support

Research suggests that magnesium intake correlates with improved lung function. Adequate magnesium levels contribute to enhanced respiratory muscle strength, potentially aiding in better respiratory efficiency and endurance, particularly beneficial for individuals with compromised lung function.

Asthma Symptom Management and Exacerbation Prevention

Incorporating magnesium into asthma management strategies holds promise in mitigating symptoms and preventing exacerbations. Studies indicate that magnesium supplementation or increased dietary intake may reduce the frequency and severity of asthma attacks, leading to improved symptom control.

Complementary Role with Bronchodilators

Magnesium's bronchodilatory effects complement conventional asthma medications, such as bronchodilators. The mineral's ability to relax airway smooth muscles may enhance the efficacy of bronchodilator medications, potentially reducing the need for higher doses of these drugs.

Part III: Magnesium in Daily Life

Chapter Seven

Understanding Magnesium Deficiency: Causes and Signs

Magnesium, an essential mineral crucial for countless bodily functions, stands as a cornerstone of optimal health. However, magnesium deficiency—a prevalent yet often undiagnosed condition—poses significant health risks and manifests through various signs and symptoms, warranting a deeper understanding of its causes and indicators.

Causes of Magnesium Deficiency

- **Inadequate Dietary Intake:** Poor dietary choices or diets lacking in magnesium-rich foods contribute to insufficient intake, exacerbating the risk of deficiency.

- **Soil Depletion:** Soil erosion and modern farming practices have led to decreased magnesium content in crops, reducing the mineral's availability in the food supply.
- **Gastrointestinal Disorders:** Conditions affecting the digestive system, such as Crohn's disease or celiac disease, can impair magnesium absorption.
- **Medications:** Certain medications, including diuretics, proton pump inhibitors, and antibiotics, may interfere with magnesium absorption or increase urinary excretion.
- **Chronic Health Conditions:** Diabetes, kidney disease, alcoholism, and aging can predispose individuals to magnesium

deficiency due to increased urinary loss or altered metabolism.

Recognizing Signs and Symptoms

- **Muscle Cramps and Spasms:** Unexplained muscle cramps, spasms, or twitching, especially in the legs, can signify magnesium deficiency.
- **Fatigue and Weakness:** Persistent fatigue, weakness, or lethargy may indicate insufficient magnesium levels impacting cellular energy production.
- **Irregular Heartbeat:** Magnesium deficiency may contribute to heart palpitations, arrhythmias, or an irregular heartbeat.
- **Mood Changes and Anxiety:** Low magnesium levels may affect

neurotransmitter function, contributing to anxiety, irritability, or mood swings.

- **Migraines or Headaches:** Individuals deficient in magnesium may experience recurrent migraines or tension headaches.
- **Insomnia or Sleep Disturbances:** Poor sleep quality, insomnia, or difficulties in falling asleep might be linked to magnesium deficiency.
- **Nausea, Loss of Appetite, or Digestive Issues:** Gastrointestinal symptoms like nausea, reduced appetite, or digestive discomfort can indicate magnesium deficiency.

Chapter Eight

Maximizing Magnesium Intake: Dietary Sources and Supplements

Ensuring adequate magnesium intake is pivotal for maintaining optimal health and addressing potential deficiencies. Exploring a range of dietary sources and supplement options offers avenues to meet the body's magnesium requirements, promoting overall well-being.

Magnesium-Rich Dietary Sources

- **Leafy Green Vegetables:** Spinach, kale, Swiss chard, and collard greens stand as excellent sources of magnesium.

- **Nuts and Seeds:** Almonds, cashews, pumpkin seeds, and sunflower seeds provide magnesium along with healthy fats and proteins.
- **Whole Grains:** Incorporating whole grains like brown rice, quinoa, and oatmeal contributes to magnesium intake.
- **Legumes:** Beans, lentils, chickpeas, and peas serve as nutritious sources of magnesium.
- **Seafood:** Some seafood options, such as salmon and mackerel, offer magnesium in addition to omega-3 fatty acids.

Fortified Foods and Other Sources

- **Fortified Cereals:** Certain breakfast cereals and fortified foods contain added magnesium, contributing to daily intake.

- **Dairy and Dairy Alternatives:** Dairy products and fortified non-dairy milk can provide magnesium.
- **Dark Chocolate:** Indulging in moderate amounts of dark chocolate (with higher cocoa content) can offer magnesium along with antioxidants.

Magnesium Supplements

- **Magnesium Citrate:** This form of magnesium is well-absorbed by the body and is commonly used to address deficiencies.
- **Magnesium Glycinate**: Known for its calming effects, magnesium glycinate is a form that may benefit individuals with anxiety or muscle tension.

- **Magnesium Oxide:** While less bioavailable, magnesium oxide is often used as a cost-effective option, but it may cause gastrointestinal discomfort in some individuals.
- **Magnesium Chloride or Lactate:** These forms are absorbed well and are often utilized for intravenous magnesium administration or as supplements.

Considerations and Dosage

- **Consultation with Healthcare Provider:** Seeking guidance from a healthcare professional can help determine appropriate dosage and supplement choice based on individual needs and health status.

- **Balanced Diet Approach:** Emphasizing a well-rounded diet rich in magnesium-containing foods remains the foundation for meeting daily magnesium requirements.
- **Supplement Dosage:** Supplement dosage may vary based on age, gender, health status, and specific health goals. It's essential to follow recommended dosages and avoid exceeding safe limits.

Chapter Nine

Enhancing Absorption: Optimizing Your Body's Utilization of Magnesium

While incorporating magnesium-rich foods and supplements is crucial, optimizing the body's absorption of this vital mineral stands as an equally essential aspect. Understanding factors that influence magnesium absorption and implementing strategies to enhance uptake ensures efficient utilization for overall health and well-being.

Pairing Magnesium with Vitamin D and Calcium

- **Vitamin D:** Vitamin D facilitates magnesium absorption by promoting the production of proteins that transport magnesium across the intestinal wall. Ensuring adequate vitamin D levels may enhance magnesium uptake.
- **Calcium-Magnesium Balance:** Maintaining a balanced ratio of calcium to magnesium aids in optimal absorption. Excessive calcium intake relative to magnesium may hinder magnesium absorption.

Dietary Factors Affecting Absorption

- **Fiber Content:** High-fiber diets can interfere with magnesium absorption as fiber binds to minerals, potentially reducing their availability. Consuming magnesium-rich foods separate from high-fiber meals may aid absorption.

- **Phytic Acid and Oxalates:** Foods high in phytic acid (found in whole grains, nuts, and seeds) and oxalates (present in spinach, beet greens) may inhibit magnesium absorption. Diversifying food sources or cooking methods can mitigate this effect.

Timing and Formulation of Supplements

- **Dividing Supplement Doses:** Splitting magnesium supplement doses throughout the day rather than taking a single large dose may enhance absorption and reduce the risk of gastrointestinal discomfort.
- **Opting for Chelated Forms:** Chelated magnesium supplements (e.g., magnesium

glycinate or citrate) are more bioavailable and better absorbed compared to other formulations.

Gut Health and Medication Interactions

- **Gut Health Optimization:** A healthy gut promotes optimal mineral absorption. Maintaining gut health through probiotics, prebiotics, and a balanced diet supports magnesium absorption.
- **Medication Consideration:** Certain medications, such as proton pump inhibitors or diuretics, may interfere with magnesium absorption. Consulting a healthcare provider regarding medication interactions is essential.

Magnesium Utilization and Exercise

- **Exercise and Magnesium Levels:** Physical activity can increase magnesium requirements due to higher utilization in energy production and muscle function. Maintaining adequate magnesium levels is crucial for active individuals.

Part IV: Lifestyle and Beyond

Chapter Ten

The Role of Magnesium in Stress Reduction and Sleep Enhancement

Magnesium, renowned for its multifaceted roles in physiological functions, exerts a profound influence on stress modulation and sleep regulation. Understanding its impact on stress reduction and sleep enhancement illuminates its significance in fostering mental well-being and promoting restful sleep.

Stress Modulation and Anxiety Alleviation

- **Neurotransmitter Regulation:** Magnesium plays a pivotal role in

regulating neurotransmitters involved in stress management, such as gamma-aminobutyric acid (GABA). GABA, an inhibitory neurotransmitter, aids in calming the nervous system, alleviating anxiety and promoting relaxation.
- **Hormonal Regulation:** Magnesium supports the regulation of stress hormones like cortisol. Adequate magnesium levels may assist in mitigating the body's stress response, reducing cortisol levels, and promoting a sense of calmness.

Sleep Quality Improvement and Insomnia Alleviation

- **Melatonin Regulation:** Magnesium contributes to the regulation of melatonin—the hormone crucial for the sleep-wake cycle. By modulating melatonin production, magnesium aids in improving sleep onset, duration, and overall sleep quality.

- **Muscle Relaxation:** Magnesium's muscle-relaxant properties contribute to physical relaxation, easing tension and promoting a more comfortable state conducive to falling asleep and staying asleep.

Magnesium and Sleep Disorders

- **Insomnia Management:** Studies suggest that magnesium supplementation may benefit individuals with insomnia by promoting relaxation and improving sleep quality.

- **Restless Leg Syndrome (RLS) Relief:** Magnesium's muscle-relaxing effects may alleviate symptoms of RLS, a condition characterized by discomfort in the legs during rest, improving sleep for affected individuals.

Stress Reduction Strategies with Magnesium

- **Stress Management Support:** Incorporating magnesium-rich foods or supplements alongside stress-reducing techniques, such as mindfulness, meditation, or relaxation exercises, may synergistically aid in stress alleviation.
- **Daily Stress Resilience:** Maintaining optimal magnesium levels through dietary

sources or supplements contributes to resilience against daily stressors, supporting mental and emotional well-being.

Chapter Eleven

Physical Activity and Magnesium: How Exercise Affects Levels

Physical activity stands as a cornerstone of overall health, yet its influence on magnesium levels and utilization within the body is an intriguing aspect worth exploring. Understanding how exercise impacts magnesium levels highlights the importance of maintaining adequate magnesium stores for optimal performance and recovery.

Magnesium Utilization during Exercise

- **Increased Metabolic Demands:** Intense physical exertion amplifies metabolic demands, leading to heightened energy production within cells. Magnesium plays a vital role in ATP synthesis—the primary energy currency—supporting muscular contractions and overall energy metabolism during exercise.

- **Electrolyte Balance**: Sweating during exercise results in electrolyte loss, including magnesium. Replenishing lost magnesium post-exercise becomes essential to restore electrolyte balance and prevent deficiencies.

Magnesium's Role in Exercise Performance

- **Muscle Function and Recovery:** Magnesium contributes to muscle function by facilitating calcium transport across cell membranes, regulating muscle contractions and relaxation. Adequate magnesium levels aid in reducing muscle cramps, spasms, and fatigue during and after exercise.
- **Energy Production Support:** Magnesium's involvement in ATP production enhances energy availability, promoting endurance and performance during prolonged physical activity.

Exercise-Induced Magnesium Loss and Requirements

- **Increased Urinary Loss**: Intense or prolonged exercise can elevate urinary excretion of magnesium, leading to increased losses. Regular physical activity may consequently raise magnesium requirements to meet the body's heightened needs.
- **Magnesium Absorption Improvement:** Regular exercise has been associated with increased magnesium absorption efficiency, potentially enhancing the body's ability to utilize available magnesium.

Strategies to Maintain Magnesium Levels

- **Balanced Diet:** Consuming magnesium-rich foods—especially after exercise—such as leafy greens, nuts, seeds, and whole grains supports replenishment of magnesium stores.
- **Supplementation Consideration:** Athletes engaging in strenuous activities may consider magnesium supplementation under the guidance of a healthcare professional to ensure adequate levels and support performance and recovery.

Chapter Twelve

Embracing the Magnesium Miracle: Actionable Steps for a Healthier Life

Harnessing the benefits of magnesium stands as a transformative journey toward enhanced health and vitality. Implementing actionable steps to incorporate magnesium-rich habits fosters a holistic approach to well-being, empowering individuals to optimize their health.

1. **Prioritize Magnesium-Rich Foods**
   - **Diversify Your Diet:** Incorporate a variety of magnesium-rich foods like leafy

greens, nuts, seeds, whole grains, legumes, and seafood into your meals.
- **Balanced Intake:** Aim for a balanced diet that provides sufficient magnesium to meet daily requirements and support bodily functions.

2. **Consider Magnesium Supplements if Needed**
- **Consultation with a Professional:** Seek guidance from a healthcare provider or nutritionist to determine if magnesium supplementation aligns with your health goals and needs.
- **Optimal Dosage:** Follow recommended dosages and choose bioavailable forms of magnesium supplements to ensure absorption.

3. **Mindful Lifestyle Practices**

- **Stress Management:** Incorporate stress-reducing techniques like meditation, yoga, deep breathing exercises, or mindfulness to alleviate stress and promote relaxation—a key element in maintaining optimal magnesium levels.
- **Regular Physical Activity:** Engage in regular exercise to support overall health, recognizing the importance of maintaining adequate magnesium levels for optimal performance and recovery.

4. **Dietary Habits and Hydration**

- **Healthy Eating Patterns:** Opt for balanced meals rich in magnesium-containing foods and consider meal planning to ensure a consistent intake of essential nutrients.

- **Hydration:** Maintain adequate hydration, as proper hydration supports mineral balance and absorption, including magnesium.

5. Health Monitoring and Professional Advice

- **Regular Check-Ups:** Schedule routine health check-ups to assess magnesium levels and overall health status, allowing for timely interventions if deficiencies are identified.
- **Professional Guidance:** Seek advice from healthcare professionals for personalized recommendations on magnesium intake, especially if managing specific health conditions or concerns.

6. Lifestyle Adjustments for Better Sleep

- **Sleep Hygiene:** Prioritize good sleep hygiene practices to improve sleep quality. Consider incorporating magnesium-rich foods or supplements to support relaxation and promote restful sleep.

Printed in Great Britain
by Amazon